# Nurse 2 Nurse

A Nurse's Comprehensive Guide to Documentation

J. Chester

For information, address J's Personal Services LLC via email.
Jarvaris Chester
jspersonalservicesllc@gmail.com

Library of Congress Cataloging -in- Publication Data has been applied for.

Paperback ISBN: 979-8-9884648-4-6

*" To all professionals in the medical field, Your dedication to caring for others is a true testament to your strength and compassion. You are making a tremendous impact on the lives of many, and your hard work and ability to put your self aside is greatly appreciated.*

*As Nurses we are expected to leave our problems at the door and give all that we can to our patients.*

*I am no acceptation, Life has definitely taught me that.. I too have my own personal struggles that I face on a daily basis but we have to continue to show up for ourselves and those that we care for..*

*Thank you for all that you do. Continue to show up for you !*

*I hope you gain something from this writing, as writing has shown to be very therapeutic for me .. "*

*Take Care ~ Jaye*

# Prologue

Welcome to this handbook that was created for nurses ! It's designed by a nurse to provide practical advice to help you thrive on the floor. As a nurse, you have worked hard to earn your licensure and are dedicated to providing the best care possible to your patients. In this handbook, I will be providing you with tips to help make your work more efficient and effective, for new and seasoned nurses alike. This handbook will also help you think about documentation in a way that protects your licensure. We know that being a nurse can be challenging, but with the right tools and mindset, you can succeed and make a difference in the lives of those you care for.

While this handbook provides practical advice and helpful tips, it's important to remember that nursing is a complex and dynamic field, and every patient and situation is unique. As a nurse, you are constantly making decisions based on your training, experience, and intuition. While the advice in this handbook can be helpful, it's ultimately up to you to use your nursing judgement to make the best decisions for your patients. So read on ... take what you find useful, and always trust your instincts and expertise.

So let's dive in and start empowering you to be the best nurse you can be!

# Content

(0.6) A space to vent

(1. 21) The importance of accurate and timely documentation

(2. 24) The legal and ethical implications of incomplete or incorrect documentation

(3. 27) Strategies for organizing and prioritizing documentation tasks

(4. 30) Best practices for charting interventions and outcomes

(5. 34) Guidelines for documenting patient assessments and vital signs

(6. 39) Techniques for writing clear and concise progress notes

(7. 43) Tips for managing electronic health records (EHRs) and using documentation software effectively

(8. 48) Strategies for addressing common documentation challenges, such as incomplete or illegible orders, conflicting information, or missing data

(9. 52) Documentation Tips

# A Space to Vent

It's not uncommon for people to have differing opinions on certain issues, and the same goes for the quote **"Nurses eat their young!"** This phrase is often used to describe the phenomenon where experienced nurses are unkind or even hostile to new or inexperienced nurses. It's understandable that this quote can be scary or unsettling for those new to the field of nursing, but it's important to note that not all nurses behave in this manner.

That being said, it's crucial for those entering the nursing profession to be aware of this issue and to take steps to prepare themselves for any challenges they may face. The transition from nursing school to the workplace can be difficult, and it's not uncommon for new nurses to feel unsure of their footing.

I see many new nurses struggling in this way, and want to impart some wisdom to help ease the transition. By acknowledging the potential for experienced nurses to be unkind, my hope is to prepare new nurses for this possibility and encourage them to be confident in their abilities. Ultimately, the goal is to create a supportive and positive environment in which all nurses can thrive.

As healthcare professionals, nurses work with people from all walks of life who are facing a variety of challenges, some nurses may be facing challenges themselves, you just may not be aware of them. It's important to remember that each patient and colleague is an individual with their own unique story and circumstances, and that we should treat them with compassion and empathy.

In addition to treating patients with grace, I want to reiterate it's also important for nurses to extend this same kindness to their colleagues and coworkers, new and seasoned. Nursing can be a stressful and demanding profession, and everyone is likely to experience challenges at some point. By choosing to approach these challenges with grace and understanding, we can create a positive and supportive environment that benefits everyone.

Ultimately, choosing grace means choosing to treat others with kindness and respect, even in difficult or challenging situations. In the nursing profession, this can mean advocating for our patients' needs, supporting our colleagues, and maintaining a positive attitude even in the face of adversity. By doing so, we can create a culture of compassion and empathy that benefits everyone involved

**Knowing about different personality types** is important in the nursing profession or any other profession for several reasons. Firstly, understanding different personalities can help nurses communicate more effectively with their patients. Patients have varying communication styles and preferences, and being able to identify and adapt to these can help build rapport and trust.

Similarly, understanding different personality types can also help nurses work more effectively with their colleagues and coworkers. By recognizing and appreciating the strengths and weaknesses of different personalities, nurses can collaborate more effectively and build stronger working relationships.

Furthermore, understanding personality types can help nurses develop self-awareness and identify areas for personal and professional growth. By understanding their own strengths and weaknesses, nurses can work to improve their communication skills, build better relationships with patients and colleagues, and become more effective caregivers.

There are many different personality types that can be found in the workplace, including but not limited to:

~ Introverts: These individuals tend to be quieter and more reserved, and may prefer to work alone or in smaller groups. They may be more reflective and thoughtful in their approach to work.why

~ Extroverts: These individuals tend to be more outgoing and sociable, and may thrive in group settings. They may enjoy brainstorming and collaborating with others.

~ Assertive personalities: These individuals are confident and self-assured, and may be more comfortable taking charge and making decisions.

~ Passive personalities: These individuals tend to be more hesitant and may avoid conflict. They may be more comfortable following the lead of others.

~ Detail-oriented personalities: These individuals are focused on the specifics and may be meticulous in their work. They may be good at spotting errors and finding solutions to problems.

~ Big-picture thinkers: These individuals tend to focus on the broader picture and may be more creative in their approach. They may be good at visualizing and strategizing.

~ Analytical personalities: These individuals are logical and methodical in their approach to work. They may be good at analyzing data and finding patterns.

~ Creative personalities: These individuals are often imaginative and may enjoy expressing themselves through art, music, or writing. They may be good at generating new ideas and solutions.

~ Collaborative personalities: These individuals enjoy working with others and may be skilled at building relationships and fostering teamwork.

~ Independent personalities: These individuals tend to work best on their own and may be more self-directed. They may be good at managing their own time and resources.

Overall, knowing about different personality types is important in the nursing profession because it can help nurses communicate more effectively, work more collaboratively, and become more self-aware. By cultivating these skills, nurses can provide better care to their patients and create a more positive and supportive work environment.

Understanding personalities in the workplace is important for several reasons:

~ Communication: Knowing the different personality types can help individuals communicate more effectively with their colleagues. For example, an extrovert may prefer to talk things out, while an introvert may need time to process information before responding.

~ Collaboration: Understanding personality types can also help individuals work more effectively in teams. For example, a detail-oriented person may complement a big-picture thinker, and an assertive personality may balance out a more passive one.

~ Conflict resolution: Recognizing different personality types can also help resolve conflicts. For example, understanding that someone is more passive may mean that they are less likely to speak up if they have an issue, so it may be necessary to solicit their feedback in a different way.

~ Employee engagement: Knowing an individual's personality type can also help with employee engagement. For example, a creative person may be more engaged if they are given opportunities to express themselves, while an analytical person may be more engaged if they are given challenging problems to solve.

## Now lets talk about "Scope of Practice"

The scope of practice in nursing refers to the specific duties, responsibilities, and actions that a nurse is authorized to perform within their professional role. The scope of practice for nurses is defined by state boards of nursing, and it varies depending on the level of nursing education and licensure.

The scope of practice for registered nurses (RNs) typically includes tasks such as administering medications, performing assessments, developing care plans, and managing patient care. Licensed practical nurses (LPNs) and licensed vocational nurses (LVNs) typically have a more limited scope of practice, which may include tasks such as taking vital signs, administering medication under the supervision of an RN, and providing basic patient care.

It's important for nurses to understand their scope of practice in order to provide safe and effective care to their patients. Nurses should be aware of the legal and ethical implications of performing tasks outside of their scope of practice, as this can put patients at risk and potentially result in disciplinary action. Additionally, nurses should be proactive in seeking out education and training opportunities to expand their knowledge and skill set within their scope of practice.

Operating within your scope of practice in nursing legally and ethically is important for several reasons:

~ Patient safety: Nursing practice is regulated to ensure patient safety. Operating outside of your scope of practice can put patients at risk of harm, as you may not have the necessary knowledge or skills to provide safe and effective care.

~ Professional integrity: As a nurse, you are responsible for upholding the ethical standards of the profession. Operating within your scope of practice ensures that you are providing care in a manner that is consistent with these standards, which helps to maintain the integrity of the profession.

~ Legal liability: Operating outside of your scope of practice can also expose you to legal liability. If you provide care that is outside of your scope of practice and a patient is harmed as a result, you may be held legally responsible.

~ Respect for other healthcare professionals: Operating within your scope of practice also helps to promote respect for other healthcare professionals. By recognizing the limits of your own expertise, you can work collaboratively with other members of the healthcare team to provide the best possible care for patients.

~ Professional development: Operating within your scope of practice also allows for professional development. By continuing to expand your knowledge and skills within your scope of practice, you can provide more advanced and specialized care to patients, which can lead to greater job satisfaction and career advancement.

Operating within your scope of practice in nursing legally and ethically is essential for ensuring patient safety, upholding professional ethics and standards, avoiding legal liability, promoting respect for other healthcare professionals, and promoting professional development.

The pandemic has brought about a lot of changes in the healthcare industry, including the rise of travel nursing and agency work.

Travel nursing involves working as a temporary nurse in different healthcare facilities across the country, often for a higher salary than traditional nursing roles.

For many nurses, travel nursing nursing has become a desirable option post-pandemic. It provides the opportunity to see new places, gain diverse experience, and earn a higher salary. Additionally, with the ongoing nursing shortage, travel nurses and agency nursing are in high demand and can often find work easily.

Travel nursing also offers flexibility, which can be a major draw for some professionals. Nurses can choose the assignments that best fit their schedule and lifestyle, whether that means working for a few weeks or several months at a time. This can be especially appealing for those who are looking for a change of pace or who want to explore new career opportunities.

While travel nursing can be a great option for some nurses, it is important to consider the potential downsides as well. Travel nurses may face challenges such as adjusting to new environments, working with unfamiliar staff, and being away from family and friends.

Agency work in nursing refers to a type of employment where nurses are contracted to work on a temporary or as-needed basis for a staffing agency, rather than being employed directly by a healthcare facility. The staffing agency is responsible for finding job assignments for the nurse and handling administrative tasks such as payroll and benefits.

Agency work can offer several benefits for nurses, such as increased flexibility and the ability to work in a variety of healthcare settings. Nurses who work for staffing agencies can choose when and where they work, and can often take extended breaks between assignments. Additionally, nurses who work for staffing agencies may have the opportunity to work in different healthcare settings, which can provide valuable experience and exposure to new clinical environments.

However, agency work can also have some drawbacks. Nurses who work for staffing agencies may have less job security than those who are employed directly by a healthcare facility, and may not have access to the same benefits such as health insurance, retirement plans, and paid time off. Additionally, agency nurses may be required to adapt quickly to new clinical environments and may not have the same level of support and resources as permanent staff.

Agency work can be a viable option for nurses who are looking for increased flexibility and variety in their work, but it's important to carefully consider the potential drawbacks and to make an informed decision about whether this type of employment is right for you.

## Travel Nurse and Agency Nurse Scope of Practice

It is extremely important for travel nurses and agency nurses to operate within their scope of practice for several reasons. Firstly, travel nurses and agency nurses are often placed in new clinical environments where they may not be familiar with the policies, procedures, and protocols of the healthcare facility. This can increase the risk of errors or adverse events if the nurse is not familiar with their scope of practice and the limitations of their role.

Secondly, travel nurses and agency nurses may be working with unfamiliar patients, and may not have access to the same level of support and resources as permanent staff. This can make it more difficult for them to identify potential risks or to seek assistance if they encounter a situation that is outside their scope of practice.

Finally, working outside of one's scope of practice can have serious legal and ethical implications, regardless of whether the nurse is a permanent staff member or a travel/agency nurse. Nurses have a duty to provide safe and effective care to their patients, and working outside of one's scope of practice can put patients at risk and potentially result in disciplinary action or legal consequences.

Overall, it's essential for all nurses, including travel and agency nurses, to be aware of their scope of practice and to operate within its boundaries. This ensures that patients receive safe and effective care, and helps to prevent potential legal and ethical issues.

As a travel nurse, it is important to work within your scope of practice and adhere to the regulations and laws of your home state. This is because each state has its own nursing practice act, which defines the scope of practice for nurses in that state. The scope of practice outlines what nurses are allowed to do and what they are not allowed to do, and it varies from state to state.

Working within your scope of practice is important because it ensures that you are providing safe and effective care to patients. It also helps to protect your nursing license and your career. If you work outside of your scope of practice, you may be at risk of violating state laws and regulations, which could result in disciplinary action or even the loss of your nursing license.

Additionally, working within your scope of practice helps to maintain patient safety and quality of care. By following the guidelines and regulations set forth by your home state, you can ensure that you are providing the best possible care to your patients, even in unfamiliar settings.

It is also important to remember that as a travel nurse, you may be working in different states with different regulations and laws. It is your responsibility to familiarize yourself with the nursing practice act of each state where you work and to work within the guidelines set forth by each state.

In summary, working within your scope of practice as a travel nurse from your home state is important for ensuring patient safety, protecting your nursing license, and upholding the laws and regulations of each state where you work.

## Peer Pressure

Birds of a feather flock together, be a gazelle.

Peer pressure in the workplace occurs when employees feel pressure from their colleagues to conform to certain behaviors, attitudes, or values. This pressure can be explicit, such as when a colleague directly encourages someone to act a certain way, or it can be implicit, such as when someone feels pressure to fit in with the group.

Peer pressure can have both positive and negative effects on the workplace. Positive peer pressure can encourage employees to work harder, be more productive, and strive for excellence. For example, if a team member consistently produces high-quality work, their colleagues may feel motivated to do the same.

However, negative peer pressure can have detrimental effects on the workplace. For example, if a group of employees engages in gossip or bullying, other employees may feel pressure to participate in these behaviors in order to fit in with the group. This can create a toxic work environment and lead to decreased job satisfaction, increased stress, and even turnover.

To address negative peer pressure in the workplace, it is important for employers to promote a culture of respect, inclusivity, and professionalism. This can be done by setting clear expectations for behavior, providing training on workplace ethics and values, and enforcing policies that prohibit bullying, harassment, or discrimination.

Individual employees can also take steps to resist negative peer pressure in the workplace. This may include setting personal boundaries, speaking up against inappropriate behavior, and seeking support from colleagues or supervisors if needed.

Overall, while peer pressure in the workplace can have both positive and negative effects, it is important to recognize and address negative peer pressure in order to promote a healthy and productive work environment.

Page left blank intentionally ..

# 1

# The importance of accurate and timely documentation

Accurate and timely documentation is crucial in nursing for several reasons:

~ Continuity of Care: Accurate documentation ensures that healthcare professionals have access to comprehensive and up-to-date information about a patient's condition, treatments, and progress. This promotes continuity of care and allows for effective communication between healthcare providers.

~ Legal and Ethical Compliance: Documentation serves as legal evidence of the care provided to patients. Accurate and timely documentation helps protect healthcare professionals by demonstrating that they followed established standards of care and fulfilled their legal and ethical responsibilities.

~ Communication and Collaboration: Documentation facilitates effective communication and collaboration among healthcare team members. It enables the sharing of important patient information, including vital signs, medications, procedures, and interventions, ensuring that everyone involved in the patient's care is well-informed.

~ Quality Improvement and Research: Documented data plays a vital role in quality improvement initiatives and research. Accurate documentation allows for the analysis of patient outcomes, identification of trends, and evaluation of the effectiveness of interventions, leading to improved healthcare practices and outcomes.

~ Reimbursement and Billing: Complete and accurate documentation is necessary for appropriate reimbursement and billing processes. It helps healthcare facilities justify the services provided, supports accurate coding, and ensures that healthcare organizations receive appropriate reimbursement for the care delivered.

In summary, accurate and timely documentation in nursing is essential for continuity of care, legal compliance, effective communication, quality improvement, research, and reimbursement purposes.

# 2

# The legal and ethical implications of incomplete or incorrect documentation

Incomplete or incorrect documentation in nursing can have significant legal and ethical implications:

~ Patient Safety and Quality of Care: Incomplete or incorrect documentation can lead to errors in patient care. It may result in miscommunication, medication errors, incorrect treatment, or delayed interventions, jeopardizing patient safety and compromising the quality of care provided.

~ Legal Liability: Inadequate documentation can expose healthcare professionals and organizations to legal liability. If there is a dispute or legal claim, incomplete or incorrect documentation may hinder the defense of healthcare providers, as it may be perceived as a lack of proper care or negligence.

~ Ethical Responsibilities: Nurses have an ethical obligation to provide accurate and comprehensive documentation. Incomplete or incorrect information can undermine trust and the ethical duty to promote patient welfare, autonomy, and beneficence. It may also impede the ability of other healthcare professionals to make informed decisions about patient care.

~ Regulatory Compliance: Healthcare facilities are subject to various regulatory requirements related to documentation. Incomplete or incorrect documentation may violate these regulations, leading to potential legal consequences, fines, or loss of licensure for healthcare professionals and organizations.

~ Reimbursement and Billing Issues: Inaccurate documentation can have financial implications. It may affect the reimbursement process, leading to denied claims, delayed payments, or allegations of fraud. Adequate documentation is necessary to support accurate coding and billing practices.

~ Research and Quality Improvement: Incomplete or incorrect documentation can compromise the integrity of research studies and quality improvement initiatives. It may result in unreliable data, hindering the ability to analyze outcomes, identify trends, and make informed decisions to improve patient care.

In summary, incomplete or incorrect documentation in nursing can have serious legal and ethical implications, including compromised patient safety, legal liability, ethical concerns, regulatory non-compliance, financial issues, and hindered research and quality improvement efforts. It is vital for nurses to prioritize accurate and comprehensive documentation to meet professional standards and ensure the best possible patient care.

# 3

# Strategies for organizing and prioritizing documentation tasks

Organizing and prioritizing documentation tasks in nursing is essential to ensure efficient and effective patient care. Here are some strategies to help with this:

~ Establish a Routine: Create a consistent routine for documentation tasks. Set aside specific times during your shift dedicated to documentation. This helps to ensure that documentation is not neglected or rushed.

~ Use Electronic Health Records (EHRs): Utilize electronic health record systems to streamline documentation processes. EHRs offer features like templates, pre-populated information, and prompts that can save time and improve accuracy. Familiarize yourself with the EHR system and take advantage of its functionalities.

~ Follow Standardized Documentation Practices: Adhere to standardized documentation practices and guidelines provided by your healthcare facility. This ensures consistency, accuracy, and compliance with legal and regulatory requirements.

~ Prioritize Based on Urgency: Prioritize documentation tasks based on the urgency and importance of the information. Focus on documenting critical patient information promptly, such as changes in condition, medications, treatments, and vital signs.

~ Utilize a Documentation Checklist: Create a checklist or use templates to guide your documentation process. This helps ensure that all necessary information is documented, minimizing the risk of missing crucial details.

~ Delegate Appropriately: Delegate non-clinical or non-complex documentation tasks to appropriate team members, such as nursing assistants or clerical staff. This allows you to focus on critical aspects of patient care while still ensuring proper documentation.

~ Avoid Duplicative Documentation: Be mindful of duplicative documentation. Streamline your entries by summarizing information rather than repeating it in multiple places. This saves time and reduces the likelihood of errors.

~ Document in Real-Time: Whenever possible, document information in real-time or as soon as feasible. This helps ensure accuracy and prevents the risk of forgetting essential details or events.

~ Collaborate and Communicate: Foster effective communication and collaboration with the healthcare team. Discuss documentation expectations, share relevant information, and clarify any ambiguities to ensure comprehensive and accurate documentation.

~ Continuous Documentation: Develop the habit of continuously documenting throughout your shift rather than leaving it all for the end. This approach reduces the risk of errors, helps maintain a clear timeline of events, and eases the workload at the end of the shift.

Remember, effective organization and prioritization of documentation tasks can help nurses provide timely, accurate, and comprehensive care while minimizing the risk of errors or omissions.

# 4

# Best practices for charting interventions and outcomes

Charting interventions and outcomes in nursing is crucial for documenting patient care and tracking progress. Here are some best practices to consider:

~ Use Clear and Objective Language: Use clear, concise, and objective language when documenting interventions and outcomes. Avoid subjective terms and vague descriptions. Be specific and provide measurable details whenever possible.

~ Document in a Timely Manner: Document interventions and outcomes as soon as feasible after providing care. This helps ensure accuracy and prevents important details from being forgotten.

~ Include Relevant Information: Include relevant details about the intervention, such as the specific actions taken, medications administered, treatments performed, or procedures carried out. Document the date, time, and your name or initials to clearly identify your involvement in the care provided.

~ Focus on Patient Response: Document the patient's response to the intervention. Describe any changes in symptoms, vital signs, or overall condition. Include objective measurements and observations to support your assessment.

~ Be Specific about Outcomes: Clearly document the outcomes of interventions. Use measurable terms to describe improvements or changes in the patient's condition, such as pain scale ratings, wound healing progress, or functional abilities. Include relevant data, such as laboratory results or diagnostic findings, if applicable.

~ Include Rationale and Collaboration: Provide the rationale behind the chosen interventions, linking them to the patient's specific needs or goals. If collaboration with other healthcare professionals occurred, document their involvement and contributions to the care plan.

~ Document Education and Patient Instructions: If patient education or instructions were provided, document the content, methods used, and the patient's understanding. Include any educational materials given or referrals made for further information or support.

~ Use Appropriate Abbreviations and Symbols: Follow your healthcare facility's approved abbreviations and symbols list when documenting interventions and outcomes. Avoid using non-standard or ambiguous abbreviations that may lead to misinterpretation.

~ Review and Validate Entries: Review your documentation entries for accuracy, completeness, and clarity. Ensure that all necessary information is included and that the documentation reflects the care provided. Validate the information with the patient to ensure accuracy and address any discrepancies.

~ Maintain Confidentiality and Privacy: Adhere to patient confidentiality and privacy guidelines when documenting interventions and outcomes. Access and share patient information only with authorized healthcare professionals involved in the patient's care.

By following these best practices, nurses can ensure that interventions and outcomes are accurately and comprehensively documented, supporting effective communication, continuity of care, and informed decision-making for the patient.

# 5

# Guidelines for documenting patient assessments and vital signs

Documenting patient assessments and vital signs accurately is crucial in nursing for effective communication and continuity of care. Here are some general guidelines to consider:

- Record Objective Findings: Document objective findings from the patient assessment using measurable terms. This includes vital signs like heart rate, blood pressure, respiratory rate, temperature, and oxygen saturation levels. Use appropriate units of measurement and specify the method or equipment used for obtaining the readings.

- Document Subjective Information: Alongside objective findings, document relevant subjective information provided by the patient, such as self-reported pain levels, symptoms, or concerns. Clearly differentiate between objective and subjective data in your documentation.

- Use Descriptive Language: Use descriptive language to accurately portray the patient's condition. Include details about the location, characteristics, severity, and duration of symptoms or abnormalities. Avoid vague or ambiguous terms.

- Document Changes and Trends: Note any changes or trends observed in the patient's assessments and vital signs over time. This helps track the patient's progress or deterioration and can assist in identifying patterns or potential issues.

- Document Assessment Techniques: Document the specific assessment techniques used, such as auscultation, palpation, inspection, or percussion. Describe your findings and any abnormalities detected during the examination.

- Include Relevant Context: Provide context for the assessments and vital signs by documenting relevant factors, such as the patient's activity level, position, or recent interventions. This helps to interpret the recorded data accurately.

- Record the Date, Time, and Your Signature: Document the date and time of each assessment and vital sign recording. Include your signature, initials, or unique identifier to verify your involvement in the documentation process.

- Document Patient Position and Environment: Note the patient's position during the assessment, whether lying, sitting, or standing. Also, document any environmental factors that may influence the patient's vital signs, such as room temperature or noise levels.

- Document Abnormal Findings and Follow-Up Actions: If any abnormal findings or concerns are identified during the assessment or vital sign measurement, document them clearly. Include any actions taken or interventions initiated in response to the findings. Follow facility protocols for reporting and escalating abnormal findings.

- Use Standardized Documentation Tools: Utilize standardized documentation tools or electronic health record systems provided by your healthcare facility. These tools often include structured templates and prompts to guide the documentation process and ensure consistency.

Remember to follow your institution's specific documentation policies and guidelines while maintaining patient confidentiality and privacy throughout the process. Accurate and comprehensive documentation of patient assessments and vital signs supports effective communication, continuity of care, and informed decision-making for the patient.

# 6

# Techniques for writing clear and concise progress notes

Writing clear and concise progress notes in nursing is important for effective communication among healthcare professionals. Here are some techniques to help you achieve this:

- Use a Structured Format: Use a structured format or template provided by your healthcare facility to guide your progress note writing. This ensures consistency and helps you include all relevant information.

- Be Objective: Write progress notes in an objective manner, focusing on factual information rather than personal opinions or judgments. Use specific and measurable terms to describe the patient's condition, progress, or response to interventions.

- Use Clear and Simple Language: Write in clear and simple language that is easily understood by a wide range of healthcare professionals. Avoid using jargon, abbreviations, or acronyms that may be unfamiliar to others.

- Focus on Key Information: Include relevant and essential information in your progress notes. Highlight important changes in the patient's condition, significant events, interventions provided, and outcomes observed. Avoid unnecessary or redundant details.

- Provide Context: Include contextual information to help readers understand the circumstances surrounding the patient's progress. This may include the patient's medical history, current treatment plan, recent procedures, or relevant social factors.

- Be Chronological: Write progress notes in a chronological order, following the timeline of the patient's care. This allows for a clear and logical flow of information, making it easier for readers to follow the patient's progress.

- Document Significantly Altered or Worsened Conditions: If there are significant changes or worsening of the patient's condition, document them promptly and clearly. Include relevant assessments, vital signs, and interventions taken in response.

- Be Brief and to the Point: Keep your progress notes concise by focusing on the essential information. Avoid unnecessary repetition or lengthy explanations. Use bullet points or numbered lists when appropriate to present information succinctly.

- Use Standardized Abbreviations: When using abbreviations, ensure they are standardized and commonly understood within your healthcare facility. Avoid using non-standard or ambiguous abbreviations that may lead to misinterpretation.

- Proofread and Edit: Before finalizing your progress notes, take the time to proofread and edit for clarity, grammar, and spelling errors. Ensure that your notes are accurate, complete, and free from any inconsistencies.

By implementing these techniques, you can write clear and concise progress notes that effectively communicate the patient's progress and facilitate continuity of care among healthcare professionals.

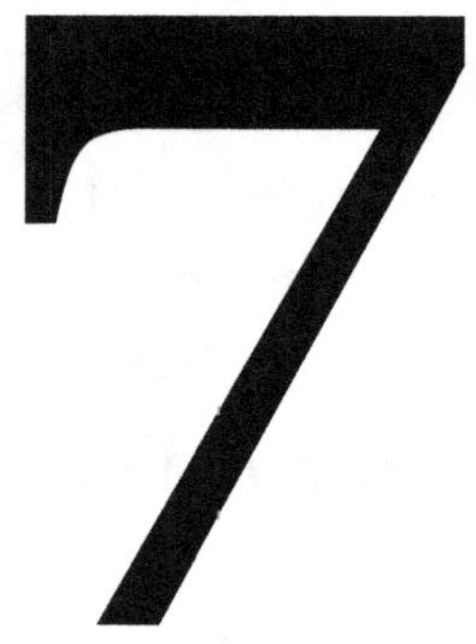

# Tips for managing electronic health records (EHRs) and using documentation software effectively

Managing electronic health records (EHRs) and using documentation software effectively in nursing can improve workflow efficiency and enhance patient care. Here are some tips to help you navigate EHRs and documentation software effectively:

- Familiarize Yourself with the EHR System: Take the time to learn and understand the functionalities, features, and navigation of your EHR system. Attend training sessions, read user manuals, or seek assistance from IT support to ensure you are proficient in using the software.

- Customize Your Workspace: Customize your EHR workspace based on your workflow and preferences. Arrange commonly used tabs, screens, or templates for easy access. Utilize features such as favorites or shortcuts to streamline your documentation process.

- Ensure Data Accuracy: Maintain accuracy in your documentation by entering information correctly and consistently. Double-check data entry, including patient demographics, medications, and vital signs, to minimize errors. Use dropdown menus, checkboxes, or pre-populated fields whenever possible to ensure consistency and accuracy.

- Utilize Templates and Macros: Take advantage of templates and macros available in your EHR system. Create or customize templates based on common documentation needs, such as assessments, progress notes, or discharge summaries. Macros can be used to automate repetitive documentation tasks, saving time and promoting consistency.

- Document in Real-Time: Aim to document patient care in real-time or as soon as feasible. This helps ensure accuracy and completeness of information. Avoid waiting until the end of the shift, as it may lead to omissions or inaccuracies.

- Maintain Patient Privacy and Confidentiality: Adhere to patient privacy and confidentiality guidelines while using EHRs. Ensure proper login/logout procedures, password protection, and adherence to HIPAA regulations. Avoid discussing patient information in public areas where screens may be visible.

- Collaborate with IT Support: Build a good relationship with your IT support team. Communicate any issues or concerns you encounter with the EHR system promptly. Provide feedback and suggestions for improvement to enhance user experience and efficiency.

- Communicate and Coordinate with the Healthcare Team: Utilize the communication features within the EHR system, such as secure messaging or shared notes, to collaborate and communicate effectively with other healthcare team members. This promotes continuity of care and reduces the risk of miscommunication.

- Stay Up-to-Date with System Updates: Keep abreast of system updates and new features introduced in your EHR software. Attend training sessions or webinars to stay informed and maximize the benefits of the system.

- Seek Continuous Improvement: Continuously evaluate and improve your documentation practices. Reflect on your workflow, identify areas for improvement, and explore additional training opportunities to enhance your EHR proficiency.

By following these tips, you can effectively manage EHRs and utilize documentation software to streamline your workflow, improve accuracy, and enhance patient care in nursing.

# 8

# Strategies for addressing common documentation challenges, such as incomplete or illegible orders, conflicting information, or missing data

Addressing common documentation challenges is crucial to ensure accurate and comprehensive patient records. Here are some strategies for addressing specific documentation challenges in nursing:

~ Incomplete or Illegible Orders:

- Communicate with the ordering healthcare provider: If you come across incomplete or illegible orders, reach out to the ordering provider for clarification or completion. Use secure messaging, phone calls, or direct communication to ensure accurate understanding and documentation.
- Seek guidance from colleagues or supervisors: Collaborate with experienced colleagues or supervisors to interpret unclear orders. Discuss the situation, gather insights, and collectively determine the best course of action.

~ Conflicting Information:

- Verify information with the patient: When faced with conflicting information, consult the patient directly to gain clarity. Ask open-ended questions, listen attentively, and validate the details to ensure accurate documentation.
- Collaborate with the healthcare team: Engage in open communication with the healthcare team to address conflicting information. Share your concerns and work together to reconcile discrepancies. Seek input from other healthcare professionals involved in the patient's care to arrive at a consensus.

~ Missing Data:

- Follow up with the relevant healthcare professionals: If you encounter missing data, reach out to the appropriate healthcare professionals, such as laboratory staff, imaging technicians, or specialists, to obtain the necessary information. Document your efforts to retrieve the missing data and any subsequent actions taken.
- Review previous documentation: Check previous documentation to see if the missing data was recorded at a different time or in a different location. Ensure that the information is not duplicated or misplaced within the electronic health record (EHR) system.

~ Implement Quality Improvement Strategies:

- Develop documentation audits: Conduct regular audits of documentation practices to identify common challenges and areas for improvement. Analyze trends, provide feedback, and offer additional training or resources to address recurring issues.
- Provide education and training: Offer ongoing education and training sessions to enhance documentation skills and promote awareness of common challenges. Cover topics such as complete and accurate documentation, effective communication, and strategies for addressing common documentation pitfalls.

~ Utilize EHR Features:

- Use decision support tools: Take advantage of decision support tools within the EHR system, such as alerts or notifications, to prompt accurate and complete documentation. These features can help prevent missing or conflicting information.

- Implement standardized documentation templates: Use standardized documentation templates provided by your healthcare facility or EHR system. These templates often prompt for essential information and can help ensure consistent and comprehensive documentation.

Remember, effective communication, collaboration, and continuous quality improvement are essential in addressing common documentation challenges. By implementing these strategies, nurses can strive for accurate, complete, and reliable documentation, ultimately enhancing patient care and safety.

# 9

# Documentation Tips

# Documentation Tips Index :


Amputation - **58**
Ascites - **60**
Behaviors - **62**
CHF (Congestive Heart Failure) - **63**
Cognitive Impairment - **65**
Congestion - **67**
Cough - **69**
Dehydration / Nutrition / Hydration - **71**
Diabetes - **73**
Dialysis - **75**
Falls - **77**
Fractures - **78**
GI Bleed - **80**
IV Fluids and Medication - **82**
Mental Status Change - **84**
MI (Myocardial Infarction) - **86**
Oxygen Use - **88**
Pain - **89**
Pressure Ulcer - **90**
Rectal Bleed - **91**
Respiratory Infection - **92**
Suctioning - **94**
Therapy Services - **96**
Thrombosis - **98**
TIA / CVA (Trans Ischemic Attack / Cerebrovascular Accident) - **99**
Total Hip / Knee Replacement - **101**
Tracheostomy Care - **102**
Tube Feeding - **104**
UTI (Urinary Tract Infection) - **106**

~~~~~~~~~~~~~~~~~~~~~~~~~~~~~~~~~~~~~~~~

This reference guide is intended to serve as a quick and user-friendly resource for clinical staff to execute specific tasks. However, please note that the guide is not comprehensive and may not reflect state-specific requirements. Therefore, it is crucial to always rely on your clinical judgement in addition to utilizing this guide.

~~~~~~~~~~~~~~~~~~~~~~~~~~~~~~~~~~~~~~~~

# Documentation

refers to the written or electronic records that document a patient's medical history, diagnosis, treatment plan, progress notes, and other relevant information regarding their healthcare. It serves as a critical tool for healthcare providers to coordinate care and make informed decisions about a patient's health.

# The Patient Record

The patient record, also known as the medical record or health record, is a comprehensive and confidential record of a patient's medical history, diagnosis, treatment plan, and other relevant information related to their healthcare. It includes a wide range of information, such as laboratory reports, imaging studies, progress notes, medication lists, and any other pertinent medical documentation. The patient record serves as a critical tool for healthcare providers to provide quality care, make informed decisions, collaborate patient centered plans and communicate with other healthcare professionals.

To ensure accurate and complete documentation, it is important to include timestamps when documenting events that were not recorded in real-time. For instance, if a patient experienced nausea with vomiting at approximately 10 am and medication was provided at 10:30 am, the documentation should reflect these time frames. Additionally, the order details should be included, such as the name of the medication, the dose, the route, the strength, and the ordering physician. It is also essential to provide a follow-up note with information on the medication's effectiveness. This will ensure that the patient's care is properly coordinated and any necessary adjustments can be made to their treatment plan.

When documenting information that was reported to you and not directly observed, it is crucial to identify the source of the information and document their exact comments. This will ensure that the information source is clear and that the documentation is accurate and complete. For instance, if a patient's family member reported that the patient experienced chest pain and shortness of breath, it is important to identify the family member as the source of the information and document their exact comments. This will help healthcare providers to make informed decisions and ensure that the patient's care is properly coordinated.

Late entry documentation should include the date that the event occurred and the words "late entry" to indicate that the documentation is being entered after the fact. For example, if an event occurred on January 1, 2023, at 9 am, and the documentation is being entered at a later time, the entry should read "late entry for 1/1/2023 at 9 am". This ensures that the medical record accurately reflects the timing of events and provides a clear indication that the documentation was entered after the fact.

# Documentation Tips

This reference guide is intended to serve as a quick and user-friendly resource for clinical staff to execute specific tasks. However, please note that the guide is not comprehensive and may not reflect state-specific requirements. Therefore, it is crucial to always rely on your clinical judgement in addition to utilizing this guide.

**Amputation** - a guide to assist in the documentation of patients with amputation site.

What to review and include in the documentation.

- Vital Signs
- Suture Line - staples, sutures and how many
- Condition of the suture line
- Edema
- Circulation
- Motion
- Sensation
- Phantom Pain
- Stump shrinker used
- Pain medication and effectiveness
- Prosthesis use
- Body image problems

When to document this information

- Every shift
- Anytime there is a change

Additional considerations
- Psych referral if needed
- Therapy referral

MD and Responsible Party must be notified along with documentation of any changes in condition, treatments, medications, refusal of treatments / medications, showers, weight loss, and any new orders, etc.

# Documentation Tips

This reference guide is intended to serve as a quick and user-friendly resource for clinical staff to execute specific tasks. However, please note that the guide is not comprehensive and may not reflect state-specific requirements. Therefore, it is crucial to always rely on your clinical judgement in addition to utilizing this guide.

**Ascites** - a guide to assist in the documentation of patients with ascites.

What to review and include in the documentation.

- Vital Signs
- Shortness of breath
- Oxygen - Refer to Oxygen documentation tip
- Measurement of abdominal girth
- Bowel Sounds
- Lung Sounds
- Pain - Refer to Pain documentation
- Medication and effectiveness
- Assistance needed with ADL's

When to document this information

- Every shift
- Anytime there is a change

Additional considerations
- Paracentesis
- Therapy services

MD and Responsible Party must be notified along with documentation of any changes in condition, treatments,

medications, refusal of treatments / medications, showers, weight loss, and any new orders, etc

# Documentation Tips

This reference guide is intended to serve as a quick and user-friendly resource for clinical staff to execute specific tasks. However, please note that the guide is not comprehensive and may not reflect state-specific requirements. Therefore, it is crucial to always rely on your clinical judgement in addition to utilizing this guide.

**Behaviors** - a guide to assist in the documentation of patients with behaviors.

What to review and include in the documentation.

- Vital Signs
- Describe the behavior exhibited
- Precipitating factors if known
- Intervention provided and response
- Any current infectious process (UTI, PNA, Cellulitis, etc.)

When to document this information

- Every shift
- Anytime there is a change to treatment
- Anytime there is a change to the patient regarding this treatment

Additional considerations

- Referral to psych services or results of current visit

MD and Responsible Party must be notified along with documentation of any changes in condition, treatments, medications, refusal of treatments / medications, showers, weight loss, and any new orders, etc.

# Documentation Tips

This reference guide is intended to serve as a quick and user-friendly resource for clinical staff to execute specific tasks. However, please note that the guide is not comprehensive and may not reflect state-specific requirements. Therefore, it is crucial to always rely on your clinical judgement in addition to utilizing this guide.

**CHF (Congestive Heart Failure)** - a guide to assist in the documentation of patients with congestive heart failure.

What to review and include in the documentation.

- Vital Signs
- Lung assessment
- Oxygen Saturation
- Use of Oxygen (continuous, PRN - as needed , NC - nasal cannula , mask, rate) - Refer to oxygen use Documentation Tips
- Edema
- Daily weights
- Chest pain and intervention
- Difficulty breathing lying flat
- Skin color to include nail beds
- Capillary refill
- Diuretic usage and outcomes
- Bipap or CPAP usage

When to document this information

- Every shift
- Anytime there is a change

Additional Considerations

- Labs
- Chest x-ray
- EKG

MD and Responsible Party must be notified along with documentation of any changes in condition, treatments, medications, refusal of treatments / medications, showers, weight loss, and any new orders, etc.

# Documentation Tips

This reference guide is intended to serve as a quick and user-friendly resource for clinical staff to execute specific tasks. However, please note that the guide is not comprehensive and may not reflect state-specific requirements. Therefore, it is crucial to always rely on your clinical judgement in addition to utilizing this guide.

**Cognitive Impairment** - a guide to assist in the documentation of patients with cognitive Impairment.

What to review and include in the documentation.

- Vital Signs
- Level of consciousness
- Level of orientation to person, place, time
- Ability to make decisions
- Ability to make needs known
- Effect on communication
- Effect on ADL's, intake and socialization
- Staff interventions with reassurance, redirection, etc.
- Anxiety
- Behaviors - refer to behaviors documentation tips

When to document this information

- Every shift
- Anytime there is a change

Additional Considerations

- Therapy Services
- Psych referral
- Dietician referral

MD and Responsible Party must be notified along with documentation of any changes in condition, treatments, medications, refusal of treatments / medications, showers, weight loss, and any new orders, etc.

# Documentation Tips

This reference guide is intended to serve as a quick and user-friendly resource for clinical staff to execute specific tasks. However, please note that the guide is not comprehensive and may not reflect state-specific requirements. Therefore, it is crucial to always rely on your clinical judgement in addition to utilizing this guide.

**Congestion** - a guide to assist in the documentation of patients with acute or chronic congestion.

What to review and include in the documentation.

- Vital Signs
- Difficulty breathing lying flat - Elevate HOB
- Lung Sounds
- Cough - Refer to cough documentation tips
- Change in level of consciousness - Refer to Mental Status Change documentation tips
- Shortness of Breath
- Dyspnea
- Pallor
- Chest Pain
- Peripheral edema
- Medication to include breathing treatment

When to document this information

- Every shift until resolved
- Anytime there is a change

Additional Considerations

- Lab
- Chest X ray

MD and Responsible Party must be notified along with documentation of any changes in condition, treatments, medications, refusal of treatments / medications, showers, weight loss, and any new orders, etc.

# Documentation Tips

This reference guide is intended to serve as a quick and user-friendly resource for clinical staff to execute specific tasks. However, please note that the guide is not comprehensive and may not reflect state-specific requirements. Therefore, it is crucial to always rely on your clinical judgement in addition to utilizing this guide.

**Cough** - a guide to assist in there documentation of patients with an acute or chronic cough

What to review and include in the documentation.

- Vital Signs
- Lung Assessment
- Respirations - labored, uneven
- Description of cough (productive, non - productive)
- Phlegm color and consistency
- Pain ir fever present
- Medications administered
- Change in mental status - refer to Mental Status documentation tips

When to document this information

- Every shift until resolved
- Anytime there is a change

Additional Considerations

- Lab
- Chest X ray

MD and Responsible Party must be notified along with documentation of any changes in condition, treatments, medications, refusal of treatments / medications, showers, weight loss, and any new orders, etc.

# Documentation Tips

This reference guide is intended to serve as a quick and user-friendly resource for clinical staff to execute specific tasks. However, please note that the guide is not comprehensive and may not reflect state-specific requirements. Therefore, it is crucial to always rely on your clinical judgement in addition to utilizing this guide.

**Dehydration / Nutrition / Hydration** - - a guide to assist in the documentation of patients with potential or actual impairments of dehydration, nutrition and / or hydration

What to review and include in the documentation.

- Vital Signs to include a finger stick if the patient is diabetic
- Appetite
- Assessment of mucous membranes
- Skin turgor
- If eyes are sunken
- Any nausea, vomiting, or diarrhea
- Fluid and meal intake
- Output
- Change in level of consciousness
- Lethargy
- Change in ADL abilities / weakness
- Interventions such as IV fluids - refer to IV medications and fluids

When to document this information

- Every shift until resolved
- Anytime there is a change to this treatment
- Anytime there is a change to the patient regarding this treatment

Additional Considerations

- Lab
- Consult with dietician
- Refer to therapy services
- Referral to dental services

MD and Responsible Party must be notified along with documentation of any changes in condition, treatments, medications, refusal of treatments / medications, showers, weight loss, and any new orders, etc.

# Documentation Tips

This reference guide is intended to serve as a quick and user-friendly resource for clinical staff to execute specific tasks. However, please note that the guide is not comprehensive and may not reflect state-specific requirements. Therefore, it is crucial to always rely on your clinical judgement in addition to utilizing this guide.

**Diabetes** - a guide to assist in the documentation of patients with the diagnosis of diabetes.

What to review and include in the documentation.

- Vital Signs to include a finger stick
- Appetite
- Oral intake
- S/S of hyper/hypoglycemia
- Level of consciousness
- Extremities with numbness or tingling
- Insulin type, dose and frequency
- Accu- Check Frequency
- Oral medications
- Compliance / noncompliance with diet
- Hypo / hyper reaction - intervention - tolerance

When to document this information

- Every shift until resolved
- Anytime there is a change

Additional Considerations

- Lab

MD and Responsible Party must be notified along with documentation of any changes in condition, treatments,

medications, refusal of treatments / medications, showers, weight loss, and any new orders, etc.

# Documentation Tips

This reference guide is intended to serve as a quick and user-friendly resource for clinical staff to execute specific tasks. However, please note that the guide is not comprehensive and may not reflect state-specific requirements. Therefore, it is crucial to always rely on your clinical judgement in addition to utilizing this guide.

**Dialysis-** a guide to assist in the documentation of patients that receives dialysis.

What to review and include in the documentation.

- Vital Signs
- Location of shunt or catheter
- Weights
- Fatigue, Headache, Pallor, Nausea
- Vomiting
- Disorientation/ safety issues
- Intake and Output
- Pruritus
- Edema
- Anorexia
- Muscle twitching
- Condition of skin around shunt or catheter
- How often dialysis is received

When to document this information

- Every shift until resolved
- Anytime there is a change to this treatment

Additional Considerations

- Psych referral if needed

MD and Responsible Party must be notified along with documentation of any changes in condition, treatments, medications, refusal of treatments / medications, showers, weight loss, and any new orders, etc.

# Documentation Tips

This reference guide is intended to serve as a quick and user-friendly resource for clinical staff to execute specific tasks. However, please note that the guide is not comprehensive and may not reflect state-specific requirements. Therefore, it is crucial to always rely on your clinical judgement in addition to utilizing this guide.

**Falls-** a guide to assist in the documentation of patients with recent or repeat falls.

What to review and include in the documentation.

- Vital Signs
- Head to toe assessment
- Range of motion and any new or existing limitations
- Any current injuries and treatment provided
- Neuro Checks if in place
- Interventions to prevent future falls
- Current risk management report if a new fall
- Any non - compliance with the interventions in place
- If a fracture is present - refer to Fracture documentation tips

When to document this information

- Every shift until resolved
- Anytime there is a change to this treatment / intervention

Additional Considerations

- Referral to therapy services or results of current visit

MD and Responsible Party must be notified along with documentation of any changes in condition, treatments, medications, refusal of treatments / medications, showers, weight loss, and any new orders, etc.

# Documentation Tips

This reference guide is intended to serve as a quick and user-friendly resource for clinical staff to execute specific tasks. However, please note that the guide is not comprehensive and may not reflect state-specific requirements. Therefore, it is crucial to always rely on your clinical judgement in addition to utilizing this guide.

**Fractures**- a guide to assist in the documentation of patients with fractures.

What to review and include in the documentation.

- Vital Signs
- Distal pulse of the fracture site
- Location of the fracture
- Type of fracture
- Cast, splint, sling
- Pain - refer to Pain documentation tips
- Pain medications
- Edema
- Weight bearing status
- Safety issues related to transfers, dressing, ambulation etc.
- If a suture line is present:

- count of staples / sutures
- Approximation
- Color
- Drainage

When to document this information

- Every shift until resolved
- Anytime there is a change

Additional Considerations

- Orthopedic follow up visits

- Is the fracture affecting ADL's, intake, sleep, socialization, communication, self image
- Psych consult if indicated

MD and Responsible Party must be notified along with documentation of any changes in condition, treatments, medications, refusal of treatments / medications, showers, weight loss, and any new orders, etc.

# Documentation Tips

This reference guide is intended to serve as a quick and user-friendly resource for clinical staff to execute specific tasks. However, please note that the guide is not comprehensive and may not reflect state-specific requirements. Therefore, it is crucial to always rely on your clinical judgement in addition to utilizing this guide.

**GI Bleed-** a guide to assist in the documentation of patients with acute or chronic GI bleed.

What to review and include in the documentation.

- Vital Signs
- Bowel Sounds
- Last bowel movement
- Color and consistency
- Any bruising
- Nose bleeds
- Rectal bleeding
- Abdominal pain
- Monitoring of sputum, emesis, stool
- Meal intake and nutritional status

When to document this information

- Every shift until resolved
- Anytime there is a change

Additional Considerations

- Lab monitoring and results

MD and Responsible Party must be notified along with documentation of any changes in condition, treatments, medications, refusal of treatments / medications, showers, weight loss, and any new orders, etc.

# Documentation Tips

This reference guide is intended to serve as a quick and user-friendly resource for clinical staff to execute specific tasks. However, please note that the guide is not comprehensive and may not reflect state-specific requirements. Therefore, it is crucial to always rely on your clinical judgement in addition to utilizing this guide.

**IV Fluids and Medication** - a guide to assist in the documentation of IV therapy.

What to review and include in the documentation.

- Vital Signs
- Type of IV (PICC, Peripheral, Central Line or Mediport)
- Location of the IV
- Type of fluid or name of medication
- Rate of fluids
- Reason for administration of fluid and /or medication
- Description of the skin at the IV site
- Description/ condition of the dressing and if it was changed
- Intake and Output
- Response to the intervention provided

When to document this information

- Every shift until resolved
- Anytime there is a change to this treatment
- Anytime there is a change to the patient regarding this treatment

Additional Considerations

- Labs

MD and Responsible Party must be notified along with documentation of any changes in condition, treatments,

medications, refusal of treatments / medications, showers, weight loss, and any new orders, etc.

# Documentation Tips

This reference guide is intended to serve as a quick and user-friendly resource for clinical staff to execute specific tasks. However, please note that the guide is not comprehensive and may not reflect state-specific requirements. Therefore, it is crucial to always rely on your clinical judgement in addition to utilizing this guide.

**Mental Status Change** - a guide to assist in the documentation of patients with an acute mental status change.

What to review and include in the documentation.

- Vital Signs
- Level of consciousness
- New or increased behaviors to include verbal aggression
- New or increased confusion
- Intake and nutrition
- Changes in incontinence
- Signs of infection
- Abdominal distention or tenderness
- Nausea, vomiting, diarrhea

When to document this information

- Every shift
- Anytime there is a change to this treatment

Additional Considerations

- Labs
- Therapy Services
- Dietician referral Labs

MD and Responsible Party must be notified along with documentation of any changes in condition, treatments,

medications, refusal of treatments / medications, showers, weight loss, and any new orders, etc.

# Documentation Tips

This reference guide is intended to serve as a quick and user-friendly resource for clinical staff to execute specific tasks. However, please note that the guide is not comprehensive and may not reflect state-specific requirements. Therefore, it is crucial to always rely on your clinical judgement in addition to utilizing this guide.

**MI (Myocardial Infarction)** - a guide to assist in the documentation of patients with an acute or chronic MI.

What to review and include in the documentation.

- Vital Signs
- Irregularities of pulse
- Toleration of therapy
- Weekly weights
- Response to medication
- Nausea / Vomiting
- Edema
- Chest Pain (recurrent / new)
- Radiating, describe (throbbing, dull, aching, etc.)
- Edema in lower extremities
- Anxiety
- Safety issues r/t weakness or depression
- Medications

When to document this information

- Every shift
- Anytime there is a change to this treatment

Additional Considerations

- Therapy Services
- Psych Referral

MD and Responsible Party must be notified along with documentation of any changes in condition, treatments, medications, refusal of treatments / medications, showers, weight loss, and any new orders, etc.

# Documentation Tips

This reference guide is intended to serve as a quick and user-friendly resource for clinical staff to execute specific tasks. However, please note that the guide is not comprehensive and may not reflect state-specific requirements. Therefore, it is crucial to always rely on your clinical judgement in addition to utilizing this guide.

**Oxygen Use** - a guide to assist in the documentation of patients that use oxygen.

What to review and include in the documentation.

- Vital Signs with O2 saturations
- Reason for oxygen use
- Route of administration
- Rate
- Respiratory rate, depth, effort
- Lung sounds
- Cough - refer to Cough documentation tips
- Activity Tolerance
- Effect on ADL
- If weaning off continuous oxygen

- Rate
- Time span tolerated
- Activity while weaning

When to document this information

- Every shift
- Anytime there is a change to this treatment

MD and Responsible Party must be notified along with documentation of any changes in condition, treatments, medications, refusal of treatments / medications, showers, weight loss, and any new orders, etc.

# Documentation Tips

This reference guide is intended to serve as a quick and user-friendly resource for clinical staff to execute specific tasks. However, please note that the guide is not comprehensive and may not reflect state-specific requirements. Therefore, it is crucial to always rely on your clinical judgement in addition to utilizing this guide.

**Pain** - a guide to assist in the documentation of patients with chronic or acute pain.

What to review and include in the documentation.

- Vital Signs
- Location of the pain
- Severity - Scale 1 - 10
- Onset
- Intensity
- Duration & Frequency
- Medication used for treatment & effectiveness

When to document this information

- Every shift until resolved
- Anytime there is a change to this treatment
- Anytime there is a change to the patient regarding this treatment

Additional considerations

- Therapy Services

MD and Responsible Party must be notified along with documentation of any changes in condition, treatments, medications, refusal of treatments / medications, showers, weight loss, and any new orders, etc.

# Documentation Tips

This reference guide is intended to serve as a quick and user-friendly resource for clinical staff to execute specific tasks. However, please note that the guide is not comprehensive and may not reflect state-specific requirements. Therefore, it is crucial to always rely on your clinical judgement in addition to utilizing this guide.

**Pressure Ulcer** - a guide to assist in the documentation of patients that have a pressure ulcer.

What to review and include in the documentation.

- Vital Signs
- Location
- Stage
- Drainage amount, color odor
- Condition of tissue around the ulcer
- Treatment tolerance
- Pain - refer to pain documentation tips
- Any physician interventions
- Weekly measurements
- Use of a specialty bed
- Nutritional interventions

When to document this information

- Every shift until resolved
- Anytime there is a change

Additional considerations

- Labs

MD and Responsible Party must be notified along with documentation of any changes in condition, treatments, medications, refusal of treatments / medications, showers, weight loss, and any new orders, etc.

# Documentation Tips

This reference guide is intended to serve as a quick and user-friendly resource for clinical staff to execute specific tasks. However, please note that the guide is not comprehensive and may not reflect state-specific requirements. Therefore, it is crucial to always rely on your clinical judgement in addition to utilizing this guide.

**Rectal Bleed** - a guide to assist in the documentation of patients with acute or chronic rectal bleeding.

What to review and include in the documentation.

- Vital Signs
- Bowel sounds
- Last bowel movement
- Color and consistency
- Any bruising to the body
- Rectal Pain
- History of hemorrhoids
- History of constipation

When to document this information

- Every shift until resolved
- Anytime there is a change

Additional considerations

- Lab monitoring and results

MD and Responsible Party must be notified along with documentation of any changes in condition, treatments, medications, refusal of treatments / medications, showers, weight loss, and any new orders, etc.

# Documentation Tips

This reference guide is intended to serve as a quick and user-friendly resource for clinical staff to execute specific tasks. However, please note that the guide is not comprehensive and may not reflect state-specific requirements. Therefore, it is crucial to always rely on your clinical judgement in addition to utilizing this guide.

**Respiratory Infection** - a guide to assist in the documentation of patients that have an acute respiratory infection.

What to review and include in the documentation.

- Vital Signs to include O2 saturation
- Oxygen Use - refer to oxygen use documentation tips
- Lung assessment
- Respiratory efforts
- Cough - refer to cough documentation tips
- Chest pain with inspiration or coughing
- New or increased sputum production
- Edema
- Change in mental status - refer to mental status change documentation tips
- Medication /Respiratory treatment

When to document this information

- Every shift until resolved
- Anytime there is a change to this treatment

Additional considerations

- Labs
- Chest X ray

MD and Responsible Party must be notified along with documentation of any changes in condition, treatments, medications, refusal of treatments / medications, showers, weight loss, and any new orders, etc.

# Documentation Tips

This reference guide is intended to serve as a quick and user-friendly resource for clinical staff to execute specific tasks. However, please note that the guide is not comprehensive and may not reflect state-specific requirements. Therefore, it is crucial to always rely on your clinical judgement in addition to utilizing this guide.

**Suctioning** - a guide to assist in the documentation of patients that have a disease process that requires suctioning.

What to review and include in the documentation.

- Vital Signs to include O2 saturation
- Type (Oral or Tracheal)
- Oxygen Use - refer to oxygen use documentation tips
- Lung Assessment
- Respiratory efforts
- Cough - refer to cough documentation tips
- Times suctioned
- Sputum amount, color and consistency
- Treatments and medications given
- Level of consciousness
- Activity Tolerance
- Effects on ADLs
- Staff interventions to assist patient

When to document this information

- Every shift
- Anytime there is a change

Additional considerations

- Labs
- Chest Xray if signs and symptoms of aspiration

MD and Responsible Party must be notified along with documentation of any changes in condition, treatments, medications, refusal of treatments / medications, showers, weight loss, and any new orders, etc.

# Documentation Tips

This reference guide is intended to serve as a quick and user-friendly resource for clinical staff to execute specific tasks. However, please note that the guide is not comprehensive and may not reflect state-specific requirements. Therefore, it is crucial to always rely on your clinical judgement in addition to utilizing this guide.

**Therapy Services** - a guide to assist in the documentation of patients in need of therapy services to include ST - Speech Therapy / OT - Occupational Therapy / PT - Physical Therapy / RT - Respiratory Therapy.

What to review and include in the documentation.

- Vital Signs
- Physical Therapy
  - Balance
  - Bed Mobility
  - Dexterity
  - Gait
  - Pain
  - Range of Motion
  - Splints, Braces
  - Transfers
- Occupational Therapy
  - Bathing
  - Dressing
  - Eating
  - Grooming
  - Other
- Speech Therapy
  - Comprehension
  - Speech / communication
  - Swallowing
  - Cognition

- Respiratory Therapy
- Activity Tolerance
- Endurance
- Tracheostomy Care
- Ventilator Status
- Attendance to therapy and compliance / non - compliance
- Level of assistance patient requires
- Progress In Therapy
- Post therapy pain or fatigue

When to document this information

- Every shift until until services are discontinued
- Anytime there is a change

Additional considerations

- Therapy Services
- Paracentesis

MD and Responsible Party must be notified along with documentation of any changes in condition, treatments, medications, refusal of treatments / medications, showers, weight loss, and any new orders, etc.

# Documentation Tips

This reference guide is intended to serve as a quick and user-friendly resource for clinical staff to execute specific tasks. However, please note that the guide is not comprehensive and may not reflect state-specific requirements. Therefore, it is crucial to always rely on your clinical judgement in addition to utilizing this guide.

**Thrombosis** - a guide to assist in the documentation of patients with a thrombus.

What to review and include in the documentation.

- Vital Signs
- Homan's Sign
- (( DO NOT MASSAGE ))
- Measurement of the extremity circumference
- Arterial pulse in the area
- Skin color and temp
- Elevate
- Edema
- Bed rest and duration
- Medication / treatment provided

When to document this information

- Every shift until resolved
- Anytime there is a change

Additional considerations

- Labs
- Ultrasound

MD and Responsible Party must be notified along with documentation of any changes in condition, treatments, medications, refusal of treatments / medications, showers, weight loss, and any new orders, etc.

# Documentation Tips

This reference guide is intended to serve as a quick and user-friendly resource for clinical staff to execute specific tasks. However, please note that the guide is not comprehensive and may not reflect state-specific requirements. Therefore, it is crucial to always rely on your clinical judgement in addition to utilizing this guide.

**TIA / CVA (Trans Ischemic Attack / Cerebrovascular Accident)** - a guide to assist in the documentation of patients with acute or chronic TIA or CVA.

What to review and include in the documentation.

- Vital Signs
- Side of body affected
- Balance issues
- Assistance needed for ADLs
- Safety measures
- Communication abilities
- Interventions to prevent contractures
- Any s/s of depression
- Changes in level of consciousness
- Swallowing issues
- Appliances required
- Ability to make needs known
- Sensory losses
- Suctioning if needed
- Choking episodes
- Edema
- Use of prosthetics or orthotics
- Neurological assessment if needed

When to document this information

- Every shift

- Anytime there is a change

Additional considerations
- Therapy Services
- Psych referral
- Dietician referral

MD and Responsible Party must be notified along with documentation of any changes in condition, treatments, medications, refusal of treatments / medications, showers, weight loss, and any new orders, etc.

# Documentation Tips

This reference guide is intended to serve as a quick and user-friendly resource for clinical staff to execute specific tasks. However, please note that the guide is not comprehensive and may not reflect state-specific requirements. Therefore, it is crucial to always rely on your clinical judgement in addition to utilizing this guide.

**Total Hip / Knee Replacement** - a guide to assist in the documentation of patients with total hip / knee replacement.

What to review and include in the documentation.

- Vital Signs
- Surgical site assessment
- Sutures or staples and amount
- Weight bearing status
- CPM frequency
- Safety issues r/t transfers and ambulation
- Pain - refer to pain documentation tips
- Pain Medications and effectiveness
- Activity tolerance

When to document this information

- Every shift
- Anytime there is a change to this treatment
- Anytime there is a change to the patient regarding this treatment

Additional considerations

- Therapy Services

MD and Responsible Party must be notified along with documentation of any changes in condition, treatments, medications, refusal of treatments / medications, showers, weight loss, and any new orders, etc.

# Documentation Tips

This reference guide is intended to serve as a quick and user-friendly resource for clinical staff to execute specific tasks. However, please note that the guide is not comprehensive and may not reflect state-specific requirements. Therefore, it is crucial to always rely on your clinical judgement in addition to utilizing this guide.

**Tracheostomy Care** - a guide to assist in the documentation of patients that require tracheostomy care.

What to review and include in the documentation.

- Vital Signs to include )2 saturation
- Oxygen use - Refer to Oxygen documentation tips
- Lung assessment
- Respiratory efforts
- Cough - Refer to cough documentation tips
- Suctioning - Refer to suctioning documentation tips
- Times suctioned
- Sputum amount, color and consistency
- Treatments and medications given
- Level of consciousness
- Activity Tolerance
- Trach site assessment
- Dressing change
- Cannula cleaning or change

When to document this information

- Every shift until resolved
- Anytime there is a change

Additional considerations

- Labs
- Chest Xray if signs and symptoms of aspiration

MD and Responsible Party must be notified along with documentation of any changes in condition, treatments, medications, refusal of treatments / medications, showers, weight loss, and any new orders, etc.

# Documentation Tips

This reference guide is intended to serve as a quick and user-friendly resource for clinical staff to execute specific tasks. However, please note that the guide is not comprehensive and may not reflect state-specific requirements. Therefore, it is crucial to always rely on your clinical judgement in addition to utilizing this guide.

**Tube Feeding** - a guide to assist in the documentation of patients that require alternative nutrition via tube feeding.

What to review and include in the documentation.

- Vital Signs
- Lung assessment
- Abdominal assessment
- Tube site assessment
- Type of tube (G, NG, J)
- Type of feeding with route and rate
- Feeding provided by gravity (bolus) or pump
- Placement checked and verified ; residual
- Amount of free water and flushes
- Treatments and medications given
- Dressing change
- Last bowel movement
- Color and consistency of stool
- Nausea and vomiting
- Skin turgor
- Weight weekly
- Oral Care
- Oral intake if pertains to patient

When to document this information

- Every shift until resolved
- Anytime there is a change

Additional considerations

- Labs
- Chest Xray if signs and symptoms of aspiration

MD and Responsible Party must be notified along with documentation of any changes in condition, treatments, medications, refusal of treatments / medications, showers, weight loss, and any new orders, etc.

# Documentation Tips

This reference guide is intended to serve as a quick and user-friendly resource for clinical staff to execute specific tasks. However, please note that the guide is not comprehensive and may not reflect state-specific requirements. Therefore, it is crucial to always rely on your clinical judgement in addition to utilizing this guide.

**UTI (Urinary Tract Infection)** - a guide to assist in the documentation of patients with a UTI.

What to review and include in the documentation.

- Vital Signs
- Frequency of urination
- Urgency
- Burning
- Color and/or odor
- New or worsened incontinence
- Nausea / Vomiting / Chills
- Pushing and acceptance of fluids
- Antibiotic therapy and tolerance to treatment
- Pain - refer to pain documentation tips
- IV intervention - refer to IV documentation tips
- Change in mental status - refer to mental status change documentation tips

When to document this information

- Every shift
- Anytime there is a change

Additional considerations

- Labs

MD and Responsible Party must be notified along with documentation of any changes in condition, treatments, medications, refusal of treatments / medications, showers, weight loss, and any new orders, etc.

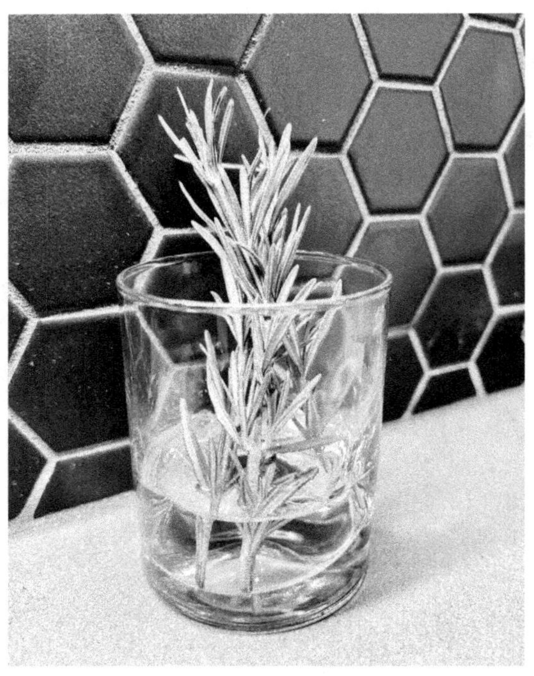

About the Author

Jaye is a passionate and experienced nurse who has dedicated his career to providing the best care possible to his patients. With quite some time of experience working in a variety of clinical settings, he has developed a deep understanding of the challenges nurses face on the floor. Through his work, he has come to recognize the critical role that documentation plays in ensuring patient safety and protecting nursing licensures. In writing this handbook, He hopes to share his knowledge and expertise with fellow nurses, empowering them to be the best they can be on the floor. Whether you're a new nurse just starting out or a seasoned professional looking for new insights, Jaye's practical advice and tips will help you excel in your role and make a difference in the lives of your patients.

www.ingramcontent.com/pod-product-compliance
Lightning Source LLC
LaVergne TN
LVHW011031110826
845149LV00015B/3371